Breath

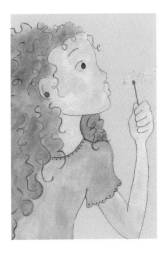

Story by
Cindy Savarda

Illustrations by
Amanda Savo

BREATH IS A GIFT,

Look inside and you will see,
take some time "to just be."

Feel your breath connect to
a spiritual fountain of peace.

When thoughts come up,
gently let them drift away.

Breathe in, breathe out,
slowly.

Inhale through the nose and
exhale fully.

Watch your belly rise
then fall with each breath.

Be still. Breathe.

Tap into the Source of
everything good.

One breath at a time.

BELIEVE IT!   BREATHE IT!!

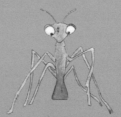

The praying mantis on
each page is a reminder
we are never alone.

This book is dedicated to my first grandchild. Gray. xoxoxo.

Grandchildren light up the world!

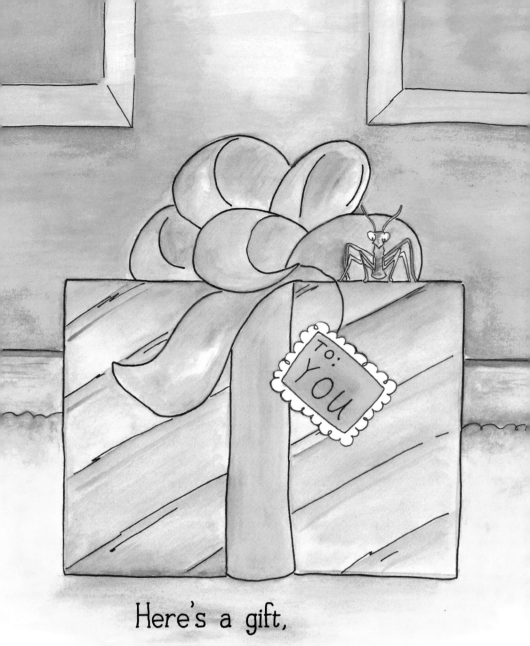

Here's a gift,

a tool for you.

Very simple,

wise and true.

Find a place,

anytime, anywhere.

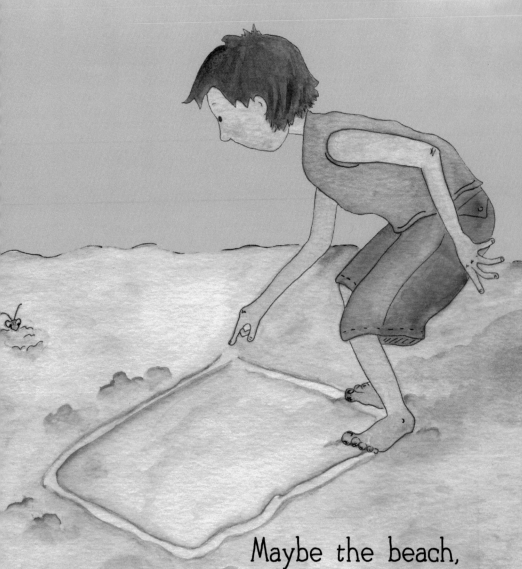

Maybe the beach,
inside your own special square.

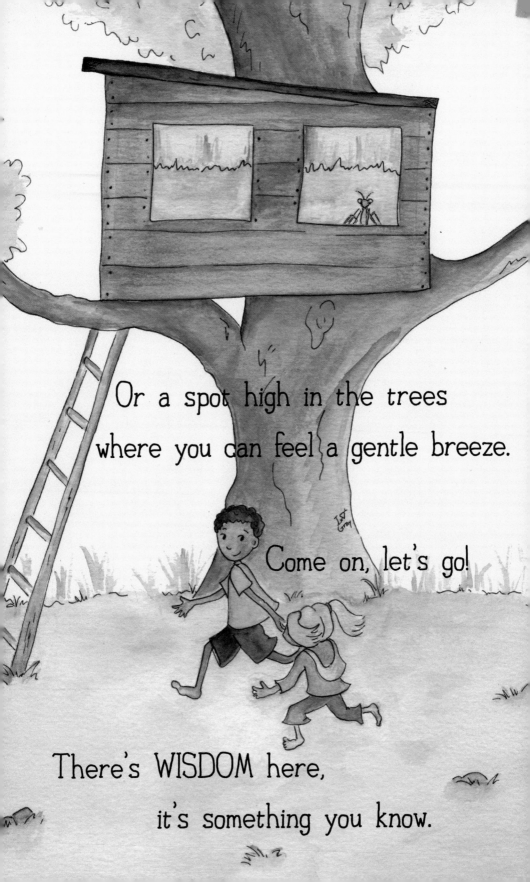

Or a spot high in the trees
where you can feel a gentle breeze.

Come on, let's go!

There's WISDOM here,
it's something you know.

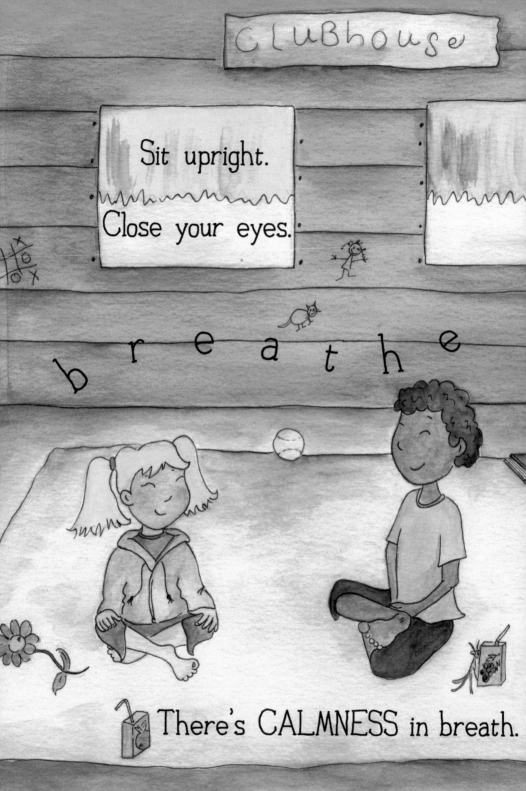

It's like the waves

in the ocean:

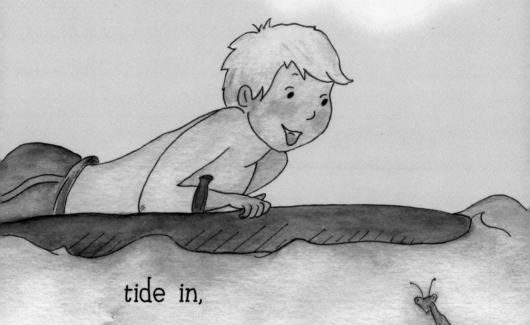

tide in,

tide out,

the pulse of the Earth.

Just do it. Don't doubt.

Sometimes you are mad,

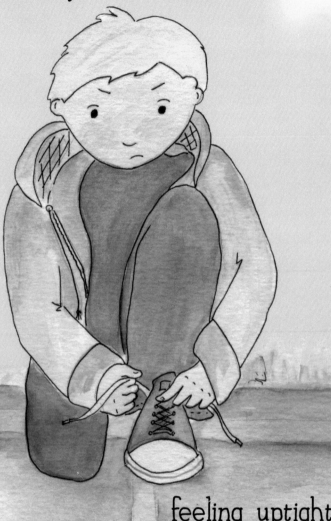

feeling uptight.

A particular situation

isn't working out just right.

It's the perfect time
to do what you know.
There is power in

B R E A T H

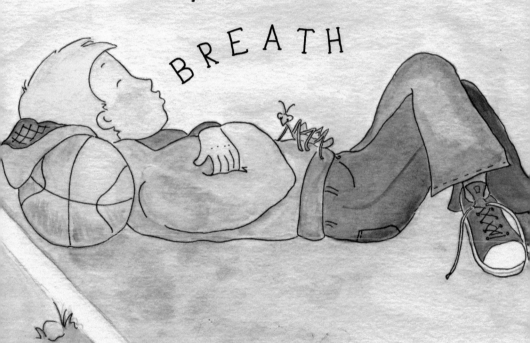

and LETTING IT GO.

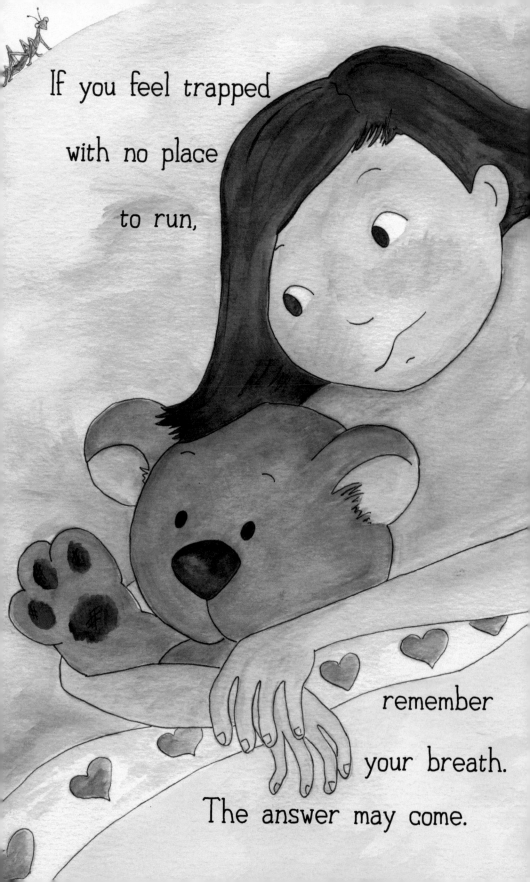

If you feel trapped
with no place
to run,

remember
your breath.
The answer may come.

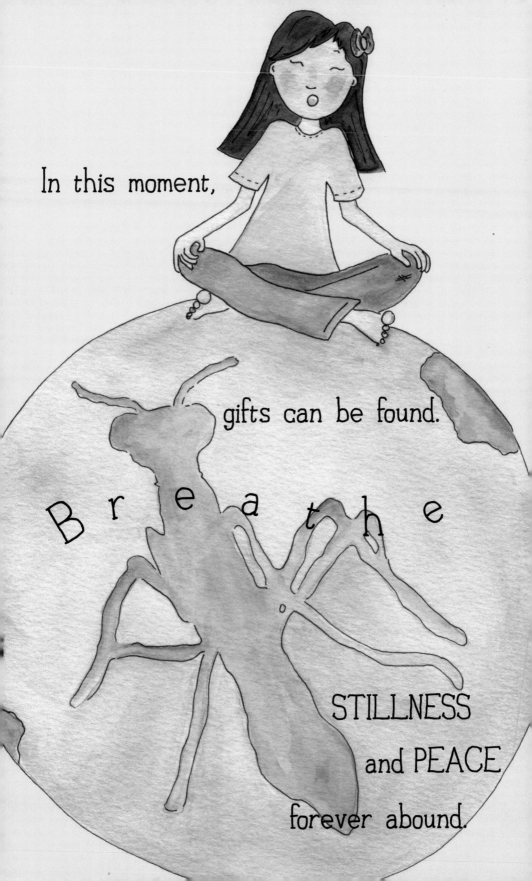

It's like magic,

I feel PEACEFUL and CALM.

Breath in,

breath out,

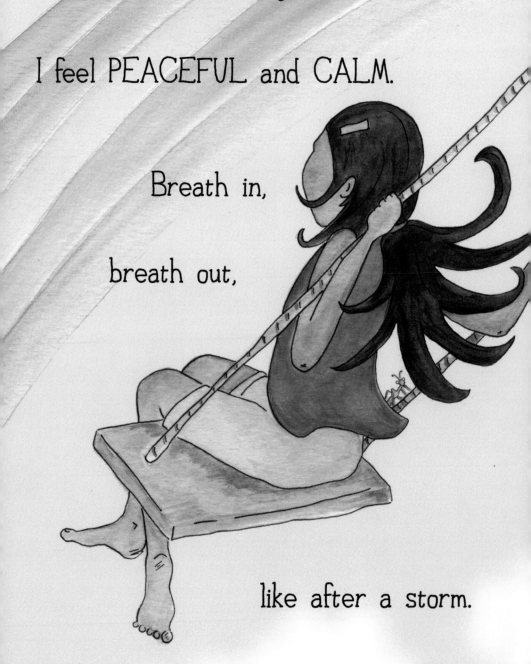

like after a storm.

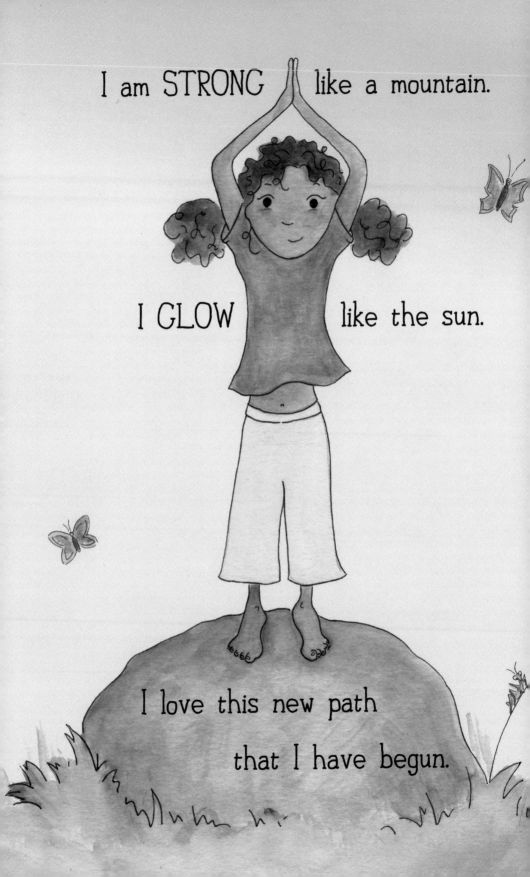

I am STRONG like a mountain.

I GLOW like the sun.

I love this new path

that I have begun.

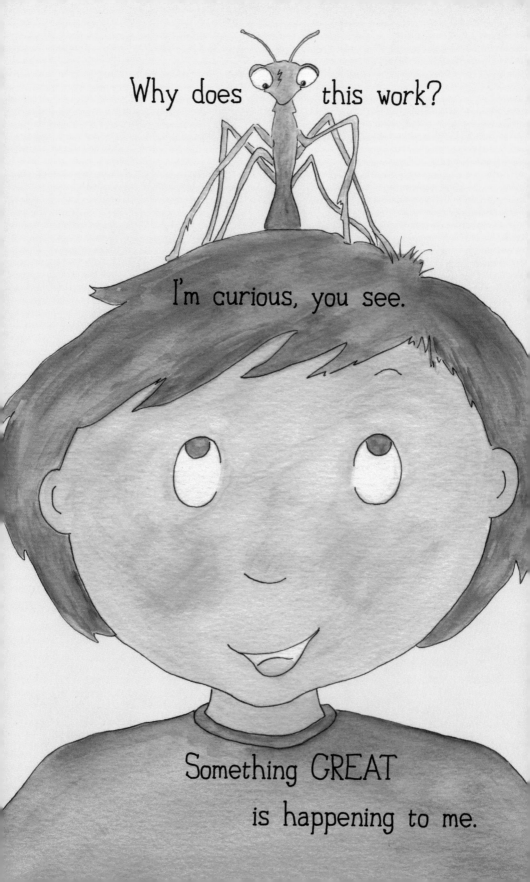

Bringing the body and mind

together this way

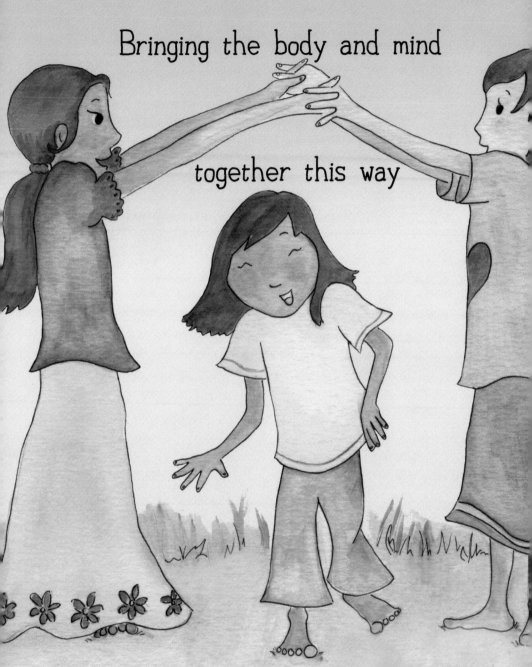

creates a bridge of UNDERSTANDING,

ENLIGHTENMENT some say.

Your breath and my breath,

where does it all go?

It keeps EVERYTHING CONNECTED

much more than we know...

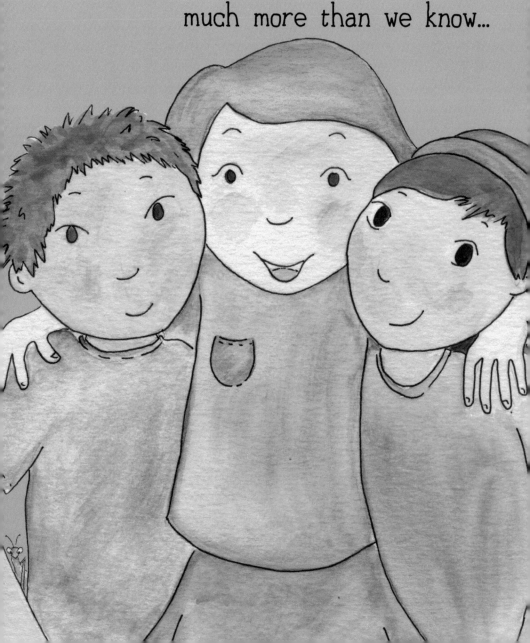

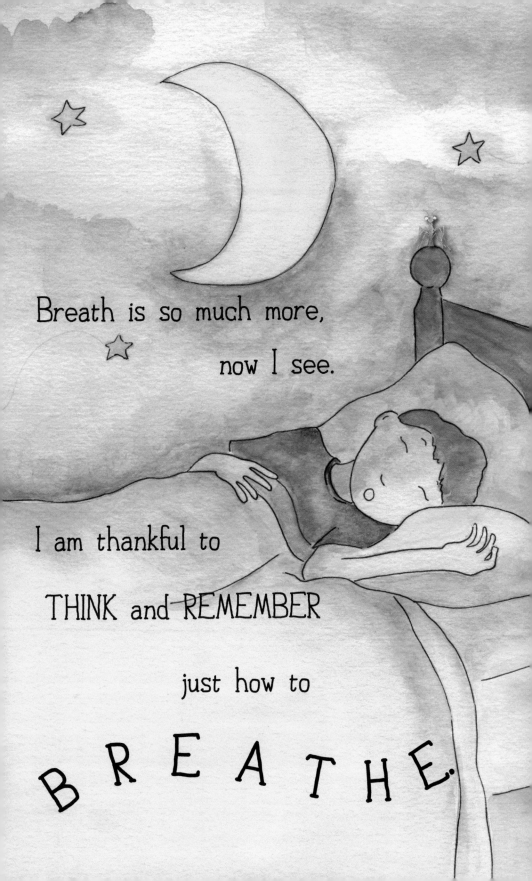

Breath is so much more,
                            now I see.

I am thankful to

THINK and REMEMBER

just how to

B R E A T H E.

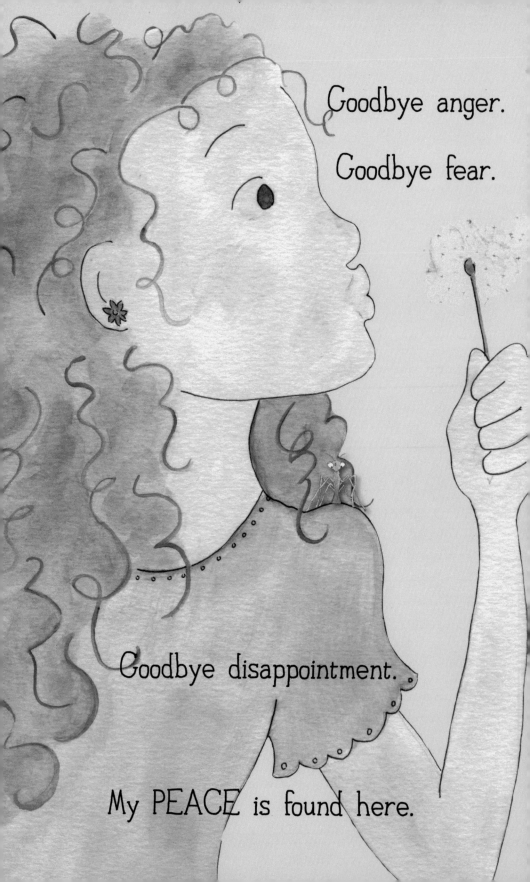

Goodbye anger.

Goodbye fear.

Goodbye disappointment.

My PEACE is found here.

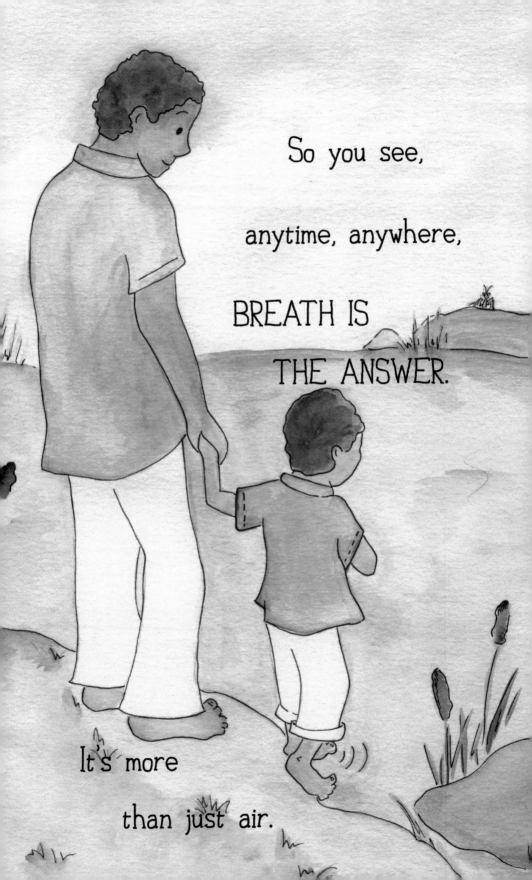

So you see,

anytime, anywhere,

BREATH IS

THE ANSWER.

It's more

than just air.

CPSIA information can be obtained
at www.ICGtesting.com
Printed in the USA
LVIC090713091112
306587LV00003B